BRANDON JAMES

The Hidden Secrets of Primal Flow

Unleashing Nature's Fitness Code

First edition

This book was professionally typeset on Reedsy.
Find out more at reedsy.com

Contents

1

Introduction: The Primal Flow Revolution: Rediscovering Nature's Fitness Code

Setting the scene:

In the bustling landscapes of the modern world, where technology reigns supreme and sedentary lifestyles have become the norm, there is an ever-growing need for a more natural and functional approach to fitness. My name is Brandon James, and I want to share with you that midst the cacophony of artificiality, a pearl of ancient wisdom calls out, beckoning us to rediscover the profound connection between our bodies and the primal rhythms of nature. This is the realm of Primal Flow, a transformative concept that transcends the confines of traditional fitness, guiding us back to the roots of movement.

Introducing the concept of Primal Flow, a journey that unearths the wisdom of our ancestral movements. Long before the gyms and exercise fads, our forebears roamed freely, navigating the untamed wilderness with grace and purpose. The legacy of their natural movements courses through our veins, waiting to be reawakened. Primal Flow is not merely an exercise routine; it is a celebration of our evolutionary heritage and a testament to the symbiotic relationship between humans and the environment. Aligning us back to our natural function and design.

In the pursuit of Primal Flow, we encounter a diverse audience of individuals who yearn for a different path in their fitness journey. They are the seekers, the dreamers, the ones who crave a deeper connection with their bodies and the world around them. Faced with the monotony and limitations of conventional fitness routines, they are ready to embrace a more holistic and authentic way of moving. Joining forces with this impassioned tribe of fitness enthusiasts, we embark on an odyssey to rediscover the timeless art of movement and unleash the hidden potential within us all.

2

CHAPTER 1: Rediscovering Our Primal Roots

Let's dive into the history of human movement, tracing its evolution from our primal ancestors to the sophisticated strides of modern humans. Delving into the annals of time, we unearth the remarkable tapestry of our movement heritage, where each step taken by our ancestors echoed the essence of survival and resilience.

Understanding the natural movements of our forebears and their relevance today, we find ourselves drawn to the ancient footprints they left behind. These natural movements, etched in the landscapes of history, serve as a beacon, guiding us back to a more instinctual way of moving. As we delve deeper, we begin to comprehend that these primal patterns are not relics of the past but enduring treasures of wisdom that hold the key to unlocking our innate physical potential.

Intriguingly, our primal instincts play a vital role in our physical well-being, mirroring the intricate harmony between humans and nature. The dance of movement is encoded in our DNA, a testament to our ancestors' profound bond with the environment they called home. As we embrace this realization, we find ourselves reconnecting with our primal selves, kindling an understanding that movement is not just an art but an integral part of the human experience. In the pages of this chapter, we uncover the significance of embracing our primal roots, transcending the boundaries of time to awaken the timeless wisdom that lies within us all.

In the depths of our being lies a primal essence, an untamed spirit that connects us to our ancient ancestors. It is a force pulsating through our veins, whispering stories of survival, resilience, and adaptability. This instinctual wisdom, buried within the sands of time, plays a vital role in our physical well-being today. As we rekindle our connection to these primal instincts, we unlock a reservoir of power, awakening dormant abilities that have withstood the test of millennia.

Our ancestors traversed rugged terrains, hunting and gathering to nourish their bodies. They moved with fluid grace, mastering the art of survival through agility and strength. Our modern lifestyles may have evolved, but the echo of those primal movements resonates within us, waiting to be rediscovered. Embracing this innate wisdom, we tap into a wellspring of physical vitality, reminding ourselves that we too are creatures of the wild, designed to thrive as one within nature's grandeur.

Amid concrete jungles and artificial comforts, our primal instincts beckon us to return to the roots of our existence. As we heed this call, our bodies respond with gratitude, unraveling the knots of sedentary living and awakening muscles long forgotten. Our physical well-being blooms as we reawaken the fierce grace of our ancestors, not confined to the iron cages of gym walls but set free in the vastness of the great outdoors. Embracing this primal heritage, we discover a symphony of movement that harmonizes body, mind, and soul - a powerful orchestra that rekindles the fire within, driving us to break boundaries and transcend limitations.

3

CHAPTER 2: The Science Behind Primal Flow

The physiological benefits of natural movement on the body and mind are nothing short of extraordinary. As we embrace the innate artistry of Primal Flow, our physical and mental realms intertwine in a harmonious symphony of well-being.

Physically, the practice of natural movement invigorates our bodies with newfound strength, flexibility, and agility. Each fluid motion, inspired by the essence of nature, challenges our muscles, bones, and joints in unique ways, enhancing their resilience and functionality. As we engage in primal patterns and dynamic exercises, our bodies undergo a metamorphosis, becoming more adaptable and prepared to handle the diverse demands of daily life.

The wonders of natural movement extend far beyond physical prowess, encompassing our mental and emotional realms as well. Engaging in mindful and purposeful movements triggers a cascade of neurochemicals, elevating our mood and reducing stress. The practice of Primal Flow becomes a gateway to tranquility, enabling us to disconnect from the chaos of modern life and reconnect with the peace that emanates from within.

Numerous studies have delved into the impact of Primal Flow movements on mobility, strength, and overall health, revealing promising results that underscore the transformative potential of this instinctive approach. In a controlled study conducted with participants of various fitness levels, researchers observed a significant improvement in joint flexibility and range of motion after just a few weeks of engaging in Primal Flow exercises. Participants reported reduced stiffness and enhanced ease of movement, a testament to the power of nature-inspired motion in enhancing mobility.

In another research endeavor, scientists examined the effects of Primal Flow on muscular strength and endurance. The findings revealed that regular engagement in animal-inspired movements, such as the Ape Reach and Bear Crawl, contributed to increased muscle activation and overall strength gains. Moreover, the dynamic nature of these exercises challenged the muscles in multiple planes of motion, fostering functional strength that better translates to real-life movements and activities. The combined benefits of improved mobility and increased strength underscore the holistic approach of Primal Flow, which not only enhances physical capabilities but also promotes a sense of well-rounded vitality and resilience.

Primal movements hold the key to unlocking a profound mind-body connection that transcends the boundaries of conventional fitness. As we immerse ourselves in the fluid grace of these instinctive motions, our minds align with the rhythm of our bodies, and a state of harmony prevails.

The deliberate and mindful nature of Primal Flow encourages us to be fully present in the moment, as we listen to our bodies' cues and respond with grace and intention. In this meditative state of movement, the distractions of the outside world fade away, leaving us with a heightened sense of self-awareness and inner peace. As we traverse the landscape of natural movements, we become attuned to the intricate dance between our physical form and our emotions, fostering a deep appreciation for the interconnectedness of our entire being. This profound mind-body connection becomes a source of empowerment, as we harness the wisdom within to navigate life's challenges with poise and confidence. The holistic benefits of Primal Flow enrich our well-being, nourishing not only our physical bodies but also our minds and spirits, propelling us on a transformation toward optimal vitality and lasting contentment.

4

CHAPTER 3: Embracing Primal Flow in Everyday Life

Integrating natural movements into our daily routines, both indoors and outdoors, is an invigorating endeavor that infuses our lives with vitality and purpose. Indoors, we can infuse our morning routines with gentle stretches inspired by animal movements like the Cat-Cow stretch or the Cobra pose. As we prepare meals in the kitchen, we can practice grounding exercises by standing barefoot on the earthy kitchen floor or experimenting with the Ape Reach to reach for items on higher shelves. Throughout the workday, we can incorporate brief movement breaks, such as the Gorilla Walk to stretch our hamstrings and release tension from sitting for prolonged periods.

Venturing outdoors presents an array of opportunities to embrace natural movements fully. During a leisurely stroll in the park, we can engage in the Traveling Beast to unleash our inner agility and connection with nature's playground. The serene ambiance of a nearby forest invites us to explore Ground Play, playfully climbing trees, and balancing on fallen logs to strengthen our core and engage our sense of adventure. When facing stairs, we can opt for the Scorpion Reach to

9

cultivate balance and flexibility, transforming mundane moments into delightful movement experiences. By creatively incorporating these natural movements into our daily routines, we seamlessly integrate the wisdom of Primal Flow into our lives, celebrating the beauty of each moment and the boundless possibilities that unfold when we embrace our innate instincts.

Primal Flow exercises offer a versatile range of movements that can be adapted to various environments, enriching our fitness journey with a touch of untamed essence. In the workplace, discreet exercises like the Underswitch can be seamlessly integrated during short breaks, fostering improved circulation and relieving the stiffness that accompanies prolonged sitting. Engaging in the Ground Play with colleagues during team-building activities invigorates our spirits and enhances camaraderie as we connect with nature's playground right outside our office doors.

If you find yourself on a nature trail, looking close enough, we can easily see the possibilities for Primal Flow expand exponentially. The Ape Reach becomes a means to embrace the towering trees, reaching for the sun-dappled canopy and strengthening our upper body. On rocky terrains, the Bear Crawl transforms into an exhilarating movement experience, testing our strength and coordination while embodying the spirit of a wild creature on the prowl. Amidst the calming sounds of a flowing river, the Frog Jump can be our playful companion, engaging our leg muscles and agility as we hop from rock to rock. Whether in the urban jungle or the wilderness, Primal Flow exercises infuse each environment with a sense of vitality, igniting our curiosity and inviting us to dance with nature's rhythm wherever our journey takes us.

To overcome common objections like time constraints and lack of expertise, we must first shift our perspective. Embrace the understanding that every moment holds full potential and possibility for movement. Incorporate brief bursts of Primal Flow exercises into our daily routines, whether it's a quick Bear Crawl in the morning or a Gorilla Walk during a lunch break. By making these practices a seamless part of our lives, we can reap the benefits of Primal Flow without compromising our busy schedules.

Furthermore, remember that Primal Flow is an instinctive and intuitive practice, accessible to all. Release the pressure to achieve perfection and focus on the joy of movement. Start with simple exercises and gradually build confidence and proficiency over time. Engage with a community, seek guidance from experienced practitioners, and share experiences with like-minded individuals. Embrace the journey of self-discovery and growth, and let go of any self-doubt. By breaking down these barriers, we open the door to a world of natural, functional, and fulfilling fitness that resonates deeply with the core of our being.

5

CHAPTER 4: Unleashing the Beast: Animal-Inspired Movements

Animal Flow exercises hold immense power, harnessing the primal essence of the animal kingdom to unleash our agility, strength, and coordination. Through these dynamic movements, we tap into the innate abilities of creatures that roam the wild, unlocking a whole new dimension of fitness. The agility of the cheetah, the strength of the bear, and the coordination of the monkey become our guiding inspirations.

With exercises like the Beast Crawl, we mimic the fluidity and grace of a wild beast, engaging multiple muscle groups to enhance our agility and mobility. The Crab Reach challenges our upper body strength and stability, replicating the movements of a crab on the shore. As we flow from one animal-inspired movement to the next, we strengthen our entire body while cultivating a profound connection with our primal instincts.

Beyond the physical gains, Animal Flow exercises immerse us in a playful and immersive fitness experience. As we explore the biomechanics of these movements, our coordination sharpens, and our body-mind connection deepens. We become more attuned to our surroundings, like the agile creatures we emulate. In this exhilarating dance with the animal kingdom, we discover a transformative path to mastering our own bodies and embodying the wild spirit within us.

The mechanics of animal-inspired movements unlock our body's innate potential as we mimic the agility and strength of various creatures. Each exercise, carefully designed to emulate animals' motions, targets specific muscle groups to enhance mobility, stability, and coordination.

For example, the Ape Reach engages our shoulder girdle and scapula, while the Bear Crawl challenges our core and improves balance. By incorporating these primal movements, we activate underutilized muscles, promoting joint health, flexibility, and overall physical resilience.

Beyond physical benefits, animal-inspired exercises evoke a sense of playfulness and connection with nature, infusing our fitness journey with joy and satisfaction. By embracing the personality of these movements, we awaken our untamed strength, redefining our perception of fitness and unlocking the hidden secrets of primal flow.

Exploring the art of creating engaging workouts with a touch of wildness using primal flow movements comes with a ton of fun. While becoming one with the freedom of the wild, we break free from conventional fitness routines and open ourselves to a world of creativity and playfulness. The key to designing captivating primal flow workouts lies in exploring a variety of animal-inspired movements.

From the agile Ape Reach to the grounded Bear Crawl, each exercise offers a unique challenge that sparks excitement and rejuvenates our love for movement and grace. By mixing and matching these primal flow movements, we create sequences that flow seamlessly, inviting us to dance with the forces of nature.

Moreover, we discover that our environment becomes our fitness playground. Whether in a lush forest or a spacious park, we unlock the potential of our surroundings to elevate our workouts to new heights. By interacting with nature's elements, we find joy in pushing our limits and immersing ourselves in a truly wild fitness experience.

Inside the appendix, you will find a carefully crafted 5-day workout plan, along with a detailed breakdown of each movement. This blueprint provides you with the tools to unleash the wild within and sculpt your body with the primal essence of nature. This can be an evolving fitness journey, where every workout brings you closer to the raw and authentic strength of our ancestors. Let the primal flow take hold, and witness the hidden secrets of nature's fitness code come to life.

Chapter 5: The Earth Beneath Our Feet: Barefooting Adventures

Barefoot training and grounding offer a profound connection between our bodies and the Earth. By engaging in barefoot training, we allow direct contact with the Earth's surface, initiating grounding or earthing. This exchange of energy has been shown to reduce stress, inflammation, and pain, while improving balance, coordination, and posture. The activation of muscles and joints in our feet during barefoot training enhances foot strength, stability, and proprioception, leading to a healthier gait and reduced risk of injuries. Embracing this practice unlocks a myriad of physical and mental health benefits, allowing us to connect with nature and improve overall well-being.

Safely transitioning to barefoot workouts requires a gradual approach to allow our feet to adapt to the new stimuli. Begin by spending short periods barefoot on natural surfaces like grass or sand, gradually increasing the duration as your feet strengthen and adjust. Focus on proper foot alignment and posture during exercises, distributing weight evenly across the feet and avoiding excessive strain on any particular area.

For those with foot-related issues, it's essential to consult a healthcare professional or a qualified fitness expert before starting a barefoot training regimen. They can provide personalized guidance and exercises to address specific concerns. Additionally, incorporating foot-strengthening exercises into your routine, such as toe curls, arch lifts, and foot massages, can help improve blood flow, foot function and alleviate sometimes seemingly unrelated problems.

By embracing barefoot workouts and taking the necessary precautions, we can unleash the innate potential of our feet and experience the raw strength of our toes and the grounding benefits that nature provides.

Connecting with nature through the soles of our feet, also known as earthing or grounding, holds a multitude of physical and mental benefits. As we walk barefoot on natural surfaces like grass, soil, or sand, our bodies establish a direct electrical connection with the Earth, facilitating the transfer of free electrons. This exchange has been found to neutralize harmful free radicals in the body, reducing inflammation and promoting faster recovery from injuries.

Grounding also plays a pivotal role in regulating our circadian rhythms and promoting better sleep. By aligning our body's internal clock with the Earth's natural cycles, we can experience improved sleep quality and wake up feeling more refreshed. Furthermore, grounding has been shown to reduce stress and promote a sense of calm and relaxation, helping to alleviate anxiety and promote emotional well-being.

Beyond the physiological benefits, connecting with nature through our feet allows us to rekindle our bond with the natural world, fostering a deeper sense of connection and appreciation for the environment. The grounding experience can provide a welcome respite from the hectic pace of modern life, offering a chance to reconnect with ourselves and the world around us in a profound and meaningful way. By embracing this simple yet powerful practice, we can harmonize our bodies with the rhythms of nature and unlock the hidden secrets of primal well-being. Remember, patience and mindful progress are key as we embark on this journey to stronger, healthier feet.

Primal Roots:
Rediscovering Harmony Through Qi-Gong Grounding

1. **Wuji Stance (Wuji Zhuang):**

Description: Stand with your feet shoulder-width apart and toes pointing slightly inward. Relax your body and bend your knees slightly, gently tuck the pelvis forward. Let your arms hang naturally by your sides with your palms facing your thighs. This foundational stance helps you connect with the earth's energy, promoting grounding and balance. Take slow deep breaths from your belly.

Maintain this posture for at least one minute.

2. **Tree Hugging (Hu Gu Gong):**

Description: Stand tall with your feet hip-width apart. Imagine embracing a tree trunk with your arms. Inhale deeply, feeling your body expand like the branches of a tree. Exhale slowly, imagining roots growing from your feet into the ground. This exercise fosters a sense of rootedness and stability.

Maintain this posture for at least one minute

3. **Bear Walking (Xiong Bu):**

Description: Take a wide stance, slightly wider than shoulder-width, and bend your knees into a low squat. Place your hands on your thighs for support. Begin walking slowly and smoothly, moving from side to side like a bear prowling through the forest. This exercise connects you with the earth's energy while promoting strength and fluidity in your movements.

Walk forward and backward for at least one minute.

4. **Earth Qigong (Di Zhou Gong):**

Description: Sit comfortably on the ground with your legs crossed. Place your palms face down on the earth beside you. Close your eyes and take slow, deep breaths, visualizing energy flowing from the earth into your body with each inhale. As you exhale, release any tension or negativity into the earth. This exercise helps you draw upon the earth's healing energy and release stagnant energy within you.

Sit for at least 2 minutes.

5. **Mountain Pose (Shan Zhuang):**

Description: Stand tall with your feet hip-width apart and your arms relaxed by your sides. Imagine yourself as a majestic mountain, rooted deep into the earth. Take slow, deep breaths, feeling the strength and stability of the mountain within you. This exercise promotes a sense of grounding and inner peace.

Maintain this posture for at least 1 minute.

Incorporating these simple Qi Gong exercises into your grounding practice amplifies your connection with nature and deepens your sense of harmony with the earth's energy. These exercises not only benefit your physical well-being but also cultivate a calm and centered mind, allowing you to tap into the profound wisdom of the earth and the universe. Let the gentle power of Qi Gong and let the earth's energy flow through you, nourishing your body, mind, and spirit.

CHAPTER 6: Primal Strength: Tapping into Nature's Forces

Developing functional strength through primal movement patterns lies at the heart of the Primal Flow approach. Unlike traditional isolated exercises that focus on specific muscle groups, primal movements engage multiple muscle groups simultaneously, mirroring the natural movements our ancestors performed for survival. By integrating these functional movements into our workouts, we cultivate strength that is applicable to real-life situations, enhancing our ability to perform daily tasks and physical challenges with ease and efficiency.

Primal movements such as crawling, jumping, and climbing demand a strong core and stable joints, fostering a well-balanced and resilient body. These dynamic exercises emphasize the importance of maintaining proper form and alignment, reducing the risk of injury while promoting joint health. Additionally, the integration of bodyweight exercises in Primal Flow workouts ensures that our muscles, tendons, and ligaments work cohesively, promoting better overall movement mechanics and preventing muscle imbalances. By embracing primal strength training, we tap into the wisdom of our ancestors and unlock the potential for functional and dynamic strength that transcends the limitations of traditional gym workouts.

Bodyweight exercises that mimic natural challenges offer a plethora of benefits that contribute to overall fitness and functional strength. For instance, the hollow body hold is an exceptional core-strengthening exercise that requires maintaining a rigid, hollow position akin to a bow. By engaging the deep abdominal muscles, hip flexors, and lower back, this exercise builds a strong and stable midsection that enhances posture and reduces the risk of lower back pain.

Another valuable bodyweight exercise is the push-up, a classic movement that targets the chest, shoulders, triceps, and core. As a functional upper-body exercise, push-ups not only build strength but also improve shoulder stability and coordination. Variations like wide grip push-ups and diamond push-ups provide unique challenges, engaging different muscle groups and promoting a well-rounded upper body development.

Exercises like the bodyweight squat and lunge work the major leg muscles, including the quads, hamstrings, and glutes, promoting lower body strength and stability. These exercises also contribute to better balance and flexibility, essential for daily activities and athletic performance. The beauty of bodyweight exercises is that they can be modified to suit individual fitness levels, making them accessible to beginners while still providing challenges for advanced practitioners. By incorporating these natural, bodyweight movements into our workouts, we tap into our evolutionary heritage and unlock the true potential of our bodies.

The synergy between Primal Flow and traditional strength training creates a harmonious blend of physical development, enabling practitioners to unleash the full potential of their bodies. While traditional strength training focuses on isolated muscle groups and heavy resistance, Primal Flow engages multiple muscle groups simultaneously, promoting functional movement patterns that mimic real-life challenges. By combining these two approaches, individuals can achieve a well-rounded and balanced physique, fortified with strength, agility, and mobility.

Primal Flow movements, such as animal-inspired exercises and ground play, enhance dynamic stability and body control, complementing traditional strength exercises like squats, dead lifts, and bench presses. Integrating both methodologies into a workout routine will surely empower individuals to not only lift heavy weights but also perform those feats with grace and precision. Moreover, the fluidity and grace derived from Primal Flow exercises enhance the mind-body connection, fostering mindfulness during strength training sessions.

The symbiotic relationship between Primal Flow and traditional strength training paves the way for optimal fitness and athletic performance. While traditional strength training builds raw strength, Primal Flow adds finesse and adaptability to movement, transcending the confines of the gym and empowering individuals to conquer physical challenges beyond their expectations. By harnessing the collective power of these two approaches, practitioners attain a holistic fitness experience, reflecting the true essence of human potential.

CHAPTER 7: From Fear to Flow: Overcoming Obstacles

Common fears often arise when venturing into unconventional exercises and embracing the world of Primal Flow. The prospect of trying new, unorthodox movements can trigger doubts about safety and effectiveness, causing apprehension in individuals. Some may worry about the risk of injury or feel uncertain about their ability to perform these unique exercises correctly. However, it's essential to recognize that Primal Flow is a customizable approach, allowing individuals to progress at their own pace and adapt movements to their current fitness level.

Addressing these fears involves a gradual and mindful introduction to Primal Flow. With proper guidance and instruction, individuals can learn the correct techniques and movement patterns, gradually building confidence in their abilities. Understanding that there is room for modification and that every journey is unique, allows individuals to navigate these fears and embark on a transformative path of self-discovery and physical empowerment. Primal Flow not only offers an opportunity to conquer these fears but also invites individuals to embrace the untamed nature of movement, unlocking their true potential and nurturing a sense of adventure within.

To ensure safe and effective movement practice in the realm of Primal Flow, a step-by-step approach is essential. First and foremost, it's crucial to start with a thorough warm-up, preparing the body for the upcoming movements and enhancing flexibility. Paying attention to proper form and alignment is paramount to avoid injury and optimize the benefits of each exercise. Begin with simple movements and progress gradually, allowing the body to adapt and strengthen over time.

As you delve into the world of Primal Flow, focus on body awareness and mindfulness. Listen to your body's cues and respect its limitations. Take breaks as needed and never push yourself beyond your comfort zone. Seek guidance from experienced coaches or instructors to receive personalized feedback and ensure you're performing movements correctly. Embrace a sense of playfulness and exploration in your practice, allowing room for creativity and intuitive movement.

Nurturing self-confidence and cultivating a fearless mindset are pivotal aspects of embracing Primal Flow with enthusiasm and determination. It's natural to encounter moments of doubt or hesitation when exploring unconventional exercises, but by recognizing these emotions and reframing them as opportunities for growth, you can build unwavering self-assurance. Embrace the journey of self-discovery, celebrating every small victory and learning from challenges along the way. Remember that progress is a personal and unique experience, and comparisons to others only hinder your potential.

To cultivate a fearless mindset, view setbacks as stepping stones rather than stumbling blocks. Embrace a mindset of resilience, where each obstacle becomes an opportunity to reassess, refine, and persevere. Approach your Primal Flow practice with a sense of adventure, curiosity, and a willingness to explore uncharted territories. By fostering self-belief and embracing the unknown, you can unlock new levels of physical, mental, and spiritual strength. In the process, you'll discover that the fearless mindset cultivated through Primal Flow transcends your fitness journey and spills over into other aspects of your life, empowering you to face challenges with courage and unwavering determination. If you following these steps, you can embrace Primal Flow safely, making it an enriching and empowering part of your fitness journey.

9

CHAPTER 8: Flow State Zen: The Art of Mindful Movement

The concept of Flow State, often referred to as being "in the zone," is a psychological state of total immersion and focus in an activity. When you enter the Flow State during Primal Movement practice, time seems to dilate, and you become fully absorbed in the present moment. Distractions fade away, and your awareness becomes razor-sharp, allowing you to perform movements with fluidity and precision. In this heightened state, you experience a profound sense of joy and fulfillment, where the practice itself becomes its own reward.

Flow State has a transformative impact on movement as it enables you to push the boundaries of your physical capabilities and tap into untapped reservoirs of potential. It is in this state of Flow that you may achieve peak performance, effortlessly moving through challenging exercises with a sense of effortlessness. The experience of Flow goes beyond just the physical aspects of movement; it also encompasses the mental and emotional realms. In the Flow State, you cultivate a deep connection between your mind and body, becoming more attuned to the subtle nuances of your movements. This heightened mind-body connection not only enhances your performance but also fosters a profound sense of mindfulness and presence during your Primal Flow practice.

The influence of Flow State on movement is truly profound. When we enter the Flow State during Primal Movement practice, time seems to disappear, and our actions flow effortlessly, as if guided by an innate wisdom. In this state, we experience a heightened focus and deep immersion in the present moment, leading to a sense of joy and fulfillment. The mind and body unite harmoniously, and our movements become fluid and instinctive, free from self-doubt and distractions. Flow State enhances the mind-body connection, allowing us to fully embody the movements and experience a state of complete engagement and satisfaction.

To access the Flow State during Primal Movement practice, we can employ several techniques. Firstly, setting a clear intention before each session provides a sense of purpose and direction, fueling our motivation to engage wholeheartedly. Secondly, finding the right balance between challenge and skill level is essential. Too easy, and we may grow bored, too difficult, and we risk becoming overwhelmed. By seeking the perfect harmony between our abilities and the challenges presented, we set the stage for the Flow State to emerge naturally.

Embracing feedback is another crucial aspect, as it fosters self-awareness and allows us to make real-time adjustments, deepening our connection to the movements. By creating an environment free from distractions and incorporating challenging sequences with a touch of playfulness, we invite the Flow State into our Primal Movement practice, elevating our fitness journey to new heights of physical and mental harmony.

Mindful physical training serves as a powerful conduit for connecting mind, body, and spirit in a harmonious union. When we engage in Primal Flow with a sense of presence and intention, each movement becomes an opportunity for self-discovery and self-awareness. Mindfulness allows us to tune into the subtle sensations within our bodies, the rhythm of our breath, and the thoughts that arise during practice. By cultivating this heightened awareness, we can better understand the intricate relationship between our physical actions and mental states. As we become attuned to the present moment, our movements flow with grace and purpose, deepening our connection to the essence of each exercise. This mindful approach not only enhances the effectiveness of our workouts but also fosters a profound sense of inner peace and spiritual alignment, transforming our Primal Movement practice into a journey of self-discovery and holistic well-being.

Qi-Gong "Enter The Flow" Movements

1. Opening the Energy Gates

Step 1: Stand with your feet shoulder-width apart and arms relaxed by your sides.

Step 2: Inhale deeply through your nose as you raise your arms slowly in front of you, palms facing upward.

Step 3: As you exhale, gently sweep your arms outward to the sides and then downwards, palms facing downward.

Step 4: Repeat this flowing motion for a few breaths, allowing the energy to flow freely through your body.

Continue for at least one minute.

2. **Cloud Hands**

Step 1: Stand with your feet shoulder-width apart and your knees slightly bent.

Step 2: Extend your right arm out in front of you, palm facing down, and your left arm to the side, palm facing up.

Step 3: Inhale deeply as you shift your weight to your right leg and move your left arm in a circular motion towards the front.

Step 4: As you exhale, shift your weight to your left leg and continue the circular motion of your left arm, bringing it back to the side.

Step 5: Repeat this flowing movement, feeling the energy flowing through your arms and your body.

Continue for at least one minute

3. **Lotus Flower**

Step 1: Stand with your feet together and your hands resting gently at your sides.

Step 2: Inhale deeply as you raise your arms above your head, palms facing each other.

Step 3: Exhale as you slowly lower your arms to your sides, visualizing the movement of a lotus flower opening and closing.

Step 4: Repeat this graceful movement, focusing on the feeling of expansion and relaxation with each breath.

Continue for at least one minute

4. Flying Crane

Step 1: Stand with your feet shoulder-width apart and your arms relaxed by your sides.

Step 2: Inhale deeply as you raise your arms in front of you, palms facing downward.

Step 3: Exhale as you open your arms to the sides, extending them outward like wings.

Step 4: Inhale again as you bring your arms back in front of you, palms facing downward.

Step 5: Exhale as you lower your arms back to your sides.

Step 6: Repeat this flowing motion, envisioning yourself as a graceful crane soaring through the sky.

Continue for at least one minute.

5. Dragon Sways Tail

Step 1: Stand with your feet shoulder-width apart and your knees slightly bent.

Step 2: Inhale deeply as you shift your weight to your right leg and extend your left arm out to the side.

Step 3: Exhale as you shift your weight to your left leg and sweep your right arm down and across your body in a curved motion, as if swaying a dragon's tail.

Step 4: Inhale again as you shift your weight back to your right leg and return your left arm to the side.

Step 5: Exhale as you shift your weight to your left leg and sweep your left arm down and across your body in a curved motion.

Step 6: Repeat this flowing movement, feeling the gentle twisting and stretching of your body.

Continue for at least one minute

Practice these Qi Gong flow movements with ease and gentleness. Allow your breath to guide the movements, and focus on cultivating a sense of harmony and flow within your body and mind. With regular practice, these movements can help you unlock the hidden secrets of Qi Gong and experience the profound benefits it offers for your overall well-being.

CHAPTER 9: Evolving Your Fitness:The Evolvish Approach

Combining modern fitness knowledge with ancestral wisdom in training presents a holistic and dynamic approach to nurturing our bodies and minds. By integrating the latest scientific findings with the timeless wisdom of our ancestors, we can tap into the full potential of our human capabilities. While modern fitness has provided us with valuable insights into physiology and exercise techniques, the wisdom of our ancestors offers a deep understanding of natural movement patterns and the interconnectedness of all living beings. The Evolvish approach, as we like to call it, encourages us to embrace the best of both worlds – drawing from modern research to inform our training methods and infusing it with the wisdom of our past to enrich our fitness journey. This harmonious blend empowers us to create personalized workouts that align with our individual needs and goals, fostering an evolutionary path towards optimal health and well-being.

We call it, "Evolvish".

The concept of Evolvish represents a groundbreaking paradigm shift in the realm of fitness, one that merges cutting-edge knowledge with the wisdom of our ancestors. At its core, the philosophy embraces the understanding that human beings have evolved over millennia, adapting to their environments and developing innate movement patterns that optimized their survival. By tapping into this ancestral wisdom, we can design personalized workouts that resonate with our bodies on a profound level, enhancing both physical and mental well-being.

In applying the principles of Evolvish, we embark on a journey of self-discovery, attuning ourselves to the unique needs and abilities of our bodies. No longer confined by rigid and standardized fitness routines, we learn to embrace our individuality, recognizing that each person's journey to optimal fitness is distinct. Evolvish empowers us to identify and address our specific weaknesses, imbalances, and strengths, allowing us to cultivate a balanced and sustainable approach to physical training. Through this mindful and intuitive process, we build a solid foundation of functional strength, improved mobility, and enhanced agility, all while honoring the natural rhythms and capacities of our bodies.

As we delve deeper into Evolvish, we discover that the key to unlocking our full potential lies in embracing the dynamic and ever-changing nature of our bodies. By continually adapting our workouts to align with our evolving needs and goals, we ensure that our progress remains consistent and gratifying. Evolvish celebrates the joy of movement and the wisdom of our ancestors, guiding us towards a deeper connection with ourselves and the natural world. With Evolvish as our compass, we journey towards a sustainable and transformative fitness experience, transcending the confines of traditional training to embrace the limitless possibilities of our human potential.

Embracing an Evolvish mindset is not solely about physical fitness but extends to optimizing our overall health and well-being. By adopting this holistic approach, we recognize the dance between of our mind, body, and spirit, working in unison to achieve a state of optimal performance and vitality. The Evolvish mindset encourages us to prioritize self-care, nourishing ourselves with wholesome nutrition, adequate rest, and stress management practices. Through this comprehensive approach, we lay the foundation for enhanced energy levels, mental clarity, and emotional balance, all of which contribute to our overall performance in every aspect of life.

As we align with the Evolvish principles, we cultivate a heightened sense of self-awareness, allowing us to better understand the signals our body sends us. This heightened awareness enables us to recognize potential imbalances and take proactive steps to address them, preventing injuries and supporting longevity in our fitness journey. By being attuned to our body's needs, we optimize our training protocols, ensuring that our workouts are effective, efficient, and tailored to our unique requirements.

Moreover, an Evolvish mindset fosters a growth-oriented perspective, embracing the idea that there is always room for improvement. Rather than viewing setbacks as failures, we perceive them as opportunities for growth and learning. This resilience and adaptability not only benefit us in the realm of fitness but also translate to our daily lives, empowering us to face challenges with confidence and courage. Through an Evolvish mindset, we continuously evolve, pushing the boundaries of what we believed possible, and unlocking the true potential that resides within us.

CHAPTER 10: Ground Play:Interacting with Nature's Playground

Imagine a world where every workout feels like an adventure, where nature becomes our playground, and the great outdoors is our natural fitness environment. Embracing nature as our gym offers an unparalleled sense of liberation and invigoration. With each step on a forest trail, each climb on a rocky terrain, and each jump over a babbling brook, we connect with the primal essence within us. The vastness of nature reminds us of our place in the universe, igniting a sense of humility and awe that fuels our determination to conquer physical challenges.

Beyond the physical benefits, immersing ourselves in nature nurtures our mental and emotional well-being. The tranquility of a quiet forest or the vastness of an open field offer solace from the chaotic modern world. Nature's beauty rejuvenates our spirit, infusing us with a profound sense of gratitude and reverence for the world around us. As we revel in the simplicity and purity of the outdoors, we rediscover our sense of wonder and curiosity, rejuvenating our mind and revitalizing our passion for life. Embracing nature's gifts as our fitness sanctuary brings us closer to our primal selves, rekindling the fire within to lead a life of vitality and purpose.

Here, we become modern-day warriors, channeling the primal instincts of our ancestors as we traverse rugged terrains, leap over boulders, and crawl through the undergrowth. The world becomes our gym, with tree branches serving as pull-up bars, rocks as stepping stones, and sandy beaches as resistance for dynamic workouts. Every landscape becomes a canvas for our imagination, and every obstacle becomes an opportunity to push our limits.

As we immerse ourselves in these creative, playful workouts, we reconnect with the joy and wonder of movement. No longer bound by the rigid structure of a traditional exercise routine, we liberate ourselves to explore our bodies' capabilities in new and exciting ways. Our senses come alive as we breathe in the fresh air, feel the earth beneath our feet, and absorb the beauty of the natural world around us. It is a journey that transcends mere physical exercise; it becomes a celebration of life and a profound connection with the environment that sustains us.

Ground Play, with its whimsical and spontaneous nature, offers far-reaching mental and emotional benefits that extend beyond the realm of physical fitness. As we engage in playful movement on the earth's canvas, a sense of childlike joy washes over us, fostering a lightheartedness that transcends the worries of daily life. The simple act of rolling on the grass, crawling through the sand, or leaping over fallen logs evokes a profound sense of freedom and carefreeness, liberating us from the stresses that burden our minds. Ground Play becomes a sanctuary for stress relief and an escape from the pressures of the modern world, where we can release pent-up energy and reconnect with the present moment.

Moreover, the immersive experience of Ground Play taps into our innate sense of curiosity and exploration. As we interact with the natural elements, our minds become attuned to the beauty and wonders of the world around us. The sights, sounds, and textures of the environment become a feast for our senses, sparking a heightened sense of awareness and mindfulness. In these moments of play, we connect with nature on a deeper level, fostering a sense of harmony and interconnectedness with the world. Ground Play becomes a moving meditation, a way to silence the noise of our thoughts and cultivate a sense of peace and tranquility within. As we embrace the mental and emotional benefits of Ground Play, we not only strengthen our bodies but also nourish our souls, finding a renewed sense of vitality and well-being in the lap of nature.

12

CONCLUSION: Beyond the Gym: A Wild Expedition to Primal Vitality

As we reach the conclusion of our transformative journey into the realm of Primal Flow, we find ourselves immersed in the profound impact of this nature-inspired approach to fitness. Throughout the chapters, we rediscovered our primal roots, unveiling the remarkable history of human movement and its evolution from our ancestors to modern humans. We delved into the physiological benefits of natural movement, witnessing how Primal Flow enhances our mobility, strength, and overall health while fostering a deep mind-body connection for improved well-being.

Embracing Primal Flow in our daily lives, we learned to seamlessly integrate natural movements into our routines, both indoors and outdoors, overcoming common objections like time constraints and lack of expertise. We unleashed the beast within through animal-inspired movements, tapping into our agility, strength, and coordination with engaging workouts that held a touch of wildness. We connected with the Earth beneath our feet, exploring the science behind barefoot training and grounding, and experiencing the benefits of nature's healing touch on our bodies and minds.

As we evolved our fitness with the Evolvish approach, we blended modern knowledge with ancestral wisdom, learning how to personalize workouts that optimized our performance and overall health. We journeyed into the state of Flow, discovering its transformative impact on our movements, and learned techniques to enter this state during Primal Movement practice, uniting our mind, body, and spirit in harmony. Embracing Ground Play in the great outdoors, we embraced creative and playful workouts, rekindling our connection with nature and reaping the mental and emotional benefits of our journey.

Reflecting on this transformative experience, we stand witness to the desired outcomes achieved by our target audience. From improved physical fitness to enhanced mental clarity and emotional well-being, Primal Flow has unlocked the potential within us, igniting a passion for mindful movement and a commitment to nature-inspired fitness. As we bid farewell to these pages, we embark on a lifelong commitment to embracing the hidden secrets of Primal Flow, unleashing nature's fitness code, and savoring the blissful harmony of mind, body, and nature. May our journey continue, forever in flow, on an evolutionary path toward optimal well-being.

In the appendix you will find:

- A description of the Primal Flow movements talked about through-out the book
- Sample workout routines for different fitness levels.
- Safety guidelines and tips for a successful Primal Flow practice.
- Additional resources and references for further exploration.

Appendix: Building Foundation: Unleashing the Beast Through Animal-Inspired Movements

Welcome to the heart of Primal Flow, where we unleash the untamed spirit within through the captivating world of Animal-Inspired Movements. Let's dive into a comprehensive Animal Flow workout plan, descriptions and instructions about the moves and focus on a new way to train for life. This is designed to strengthen your body, ignite your creativity, and awaken your primal instincts.

Animal Flow Exercises:

1. Beast Crawl: Start in a quadruped position with hands and feet on the ground. Crawl forward with opposite limbs moving simultaneously, maintaining a low, controlled stance.

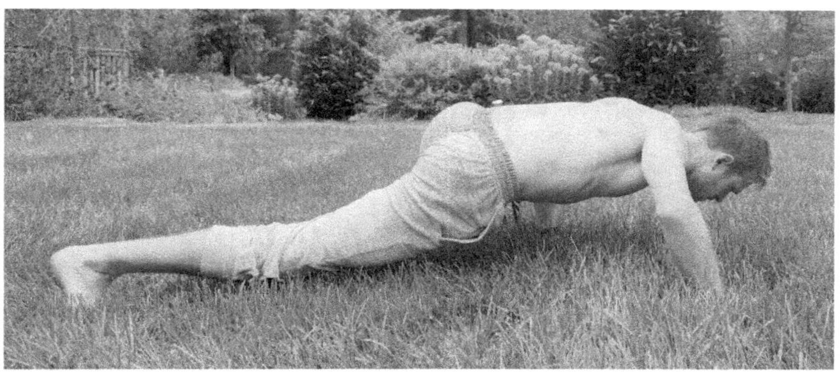

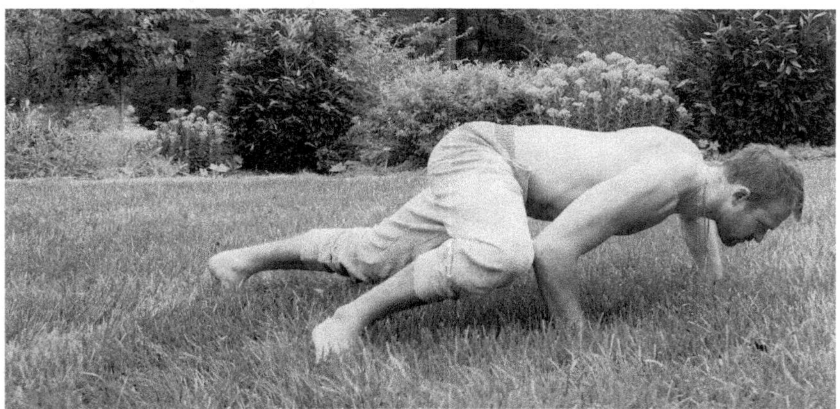

2. Crab Reach: Sit on the floor with hands and feet flat, fingers pointing backward. Lift your hips up and reach one arm overhead, following your hand with your gaze. Alternate sides.

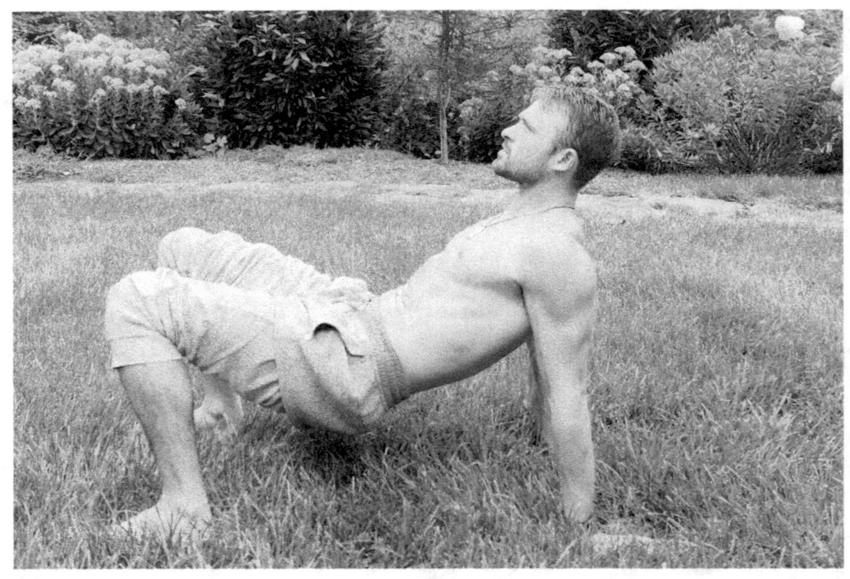

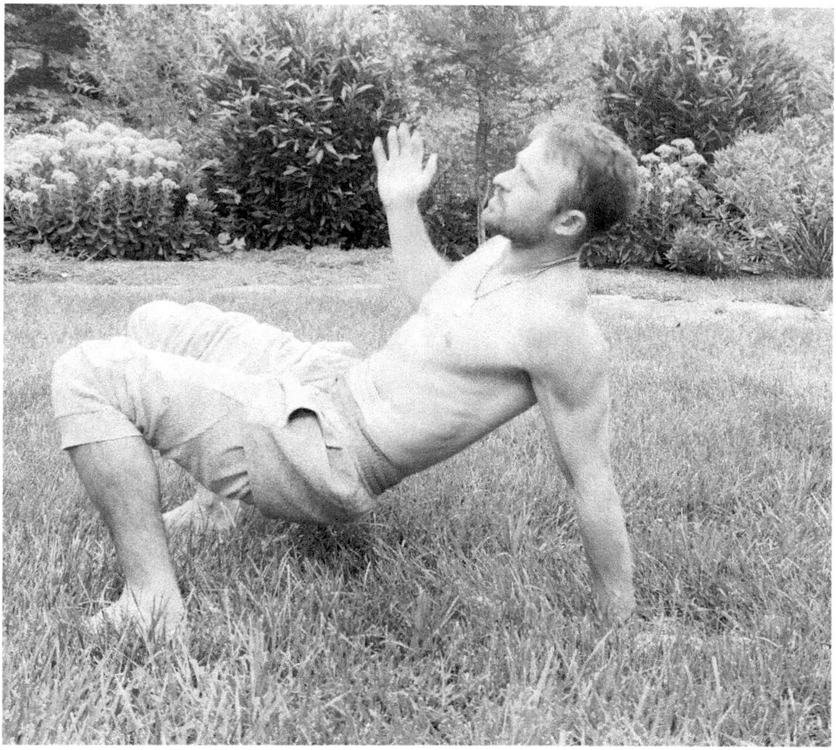

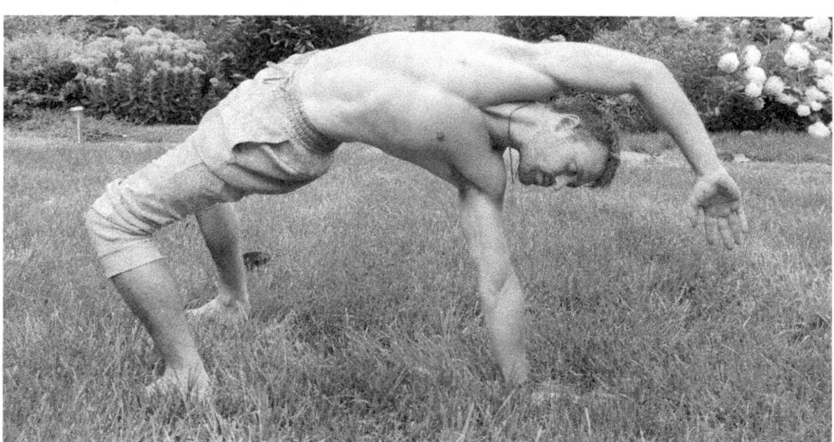

3. Ape Reach: Stand with feet wider than shoulder-width apart, toes pointed outward. Squat down and with the back of your palms facing each other, round your back and reach forward with fingertips pointed, exhaling. On the inhale, lift your chest, raise onto your toes, and bring both of your arms our straight, squeezing your shoulder blades.

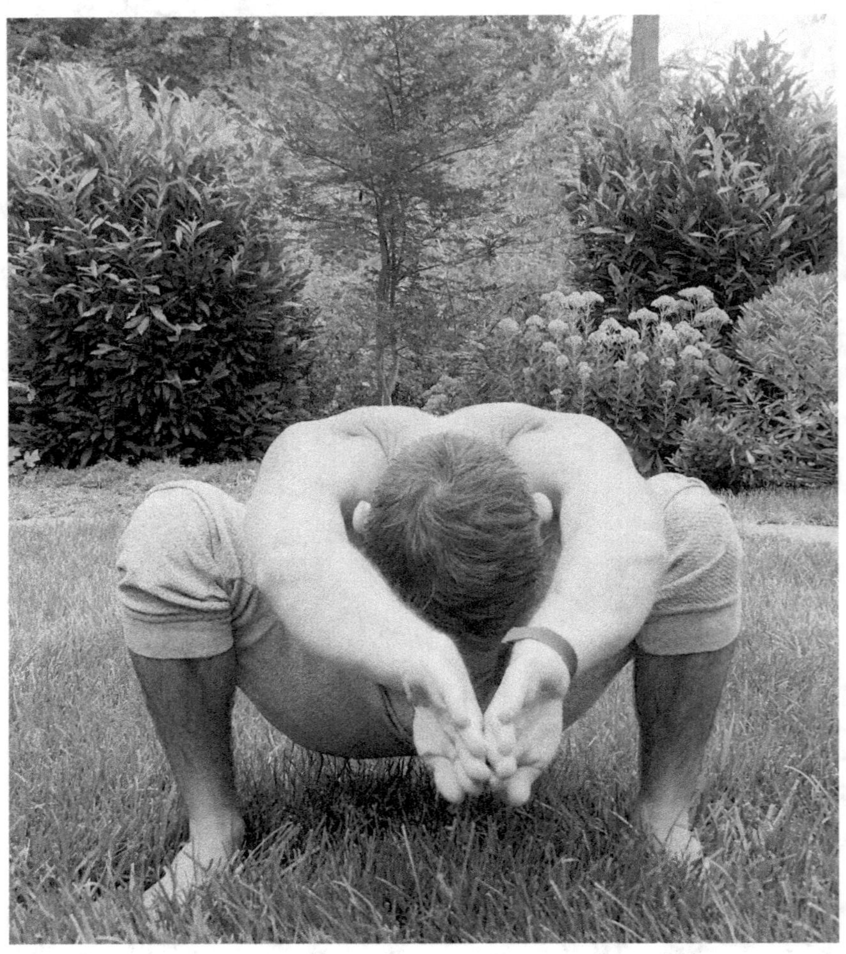

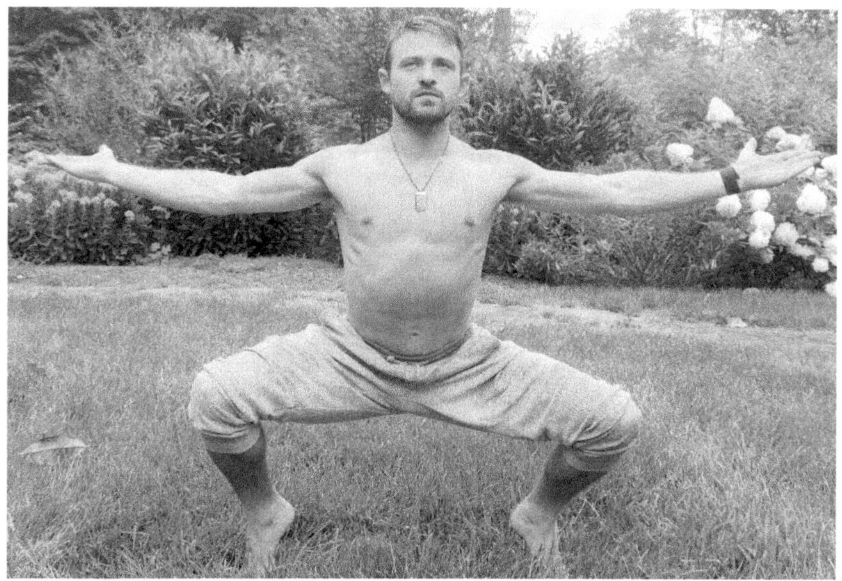

4. Bear Crawl: Begin in a quadruped position, then lift knees a few inches off the ground and no further than under your belly button. Crawl forward with opposite limbs moving together, keeping hips square and core engaged.

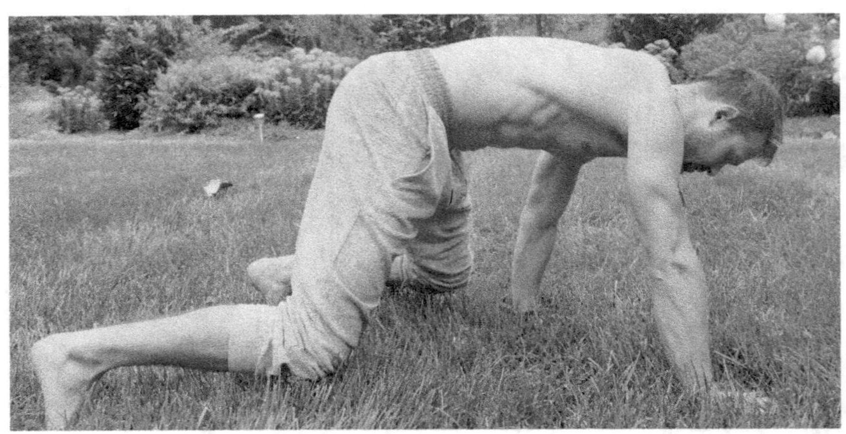

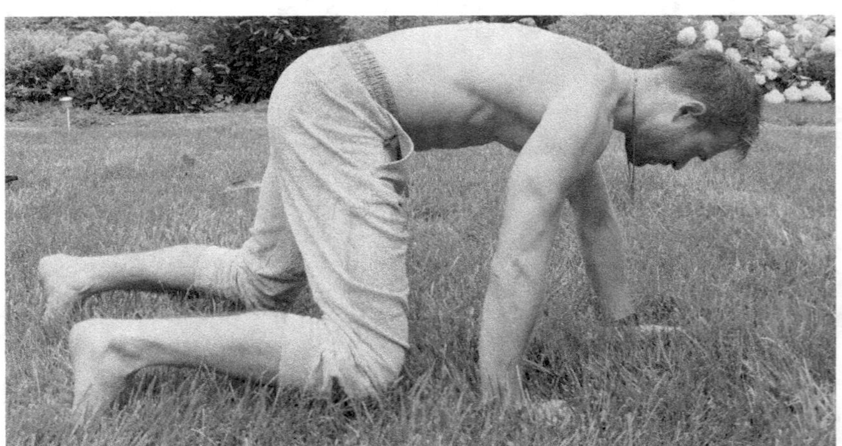

5. Underswitch: Start in a crab position and then lift one hand and foot off the ground, bringing your leg underneath your body and arm over your body to the opposite side, switching sides smoothly.

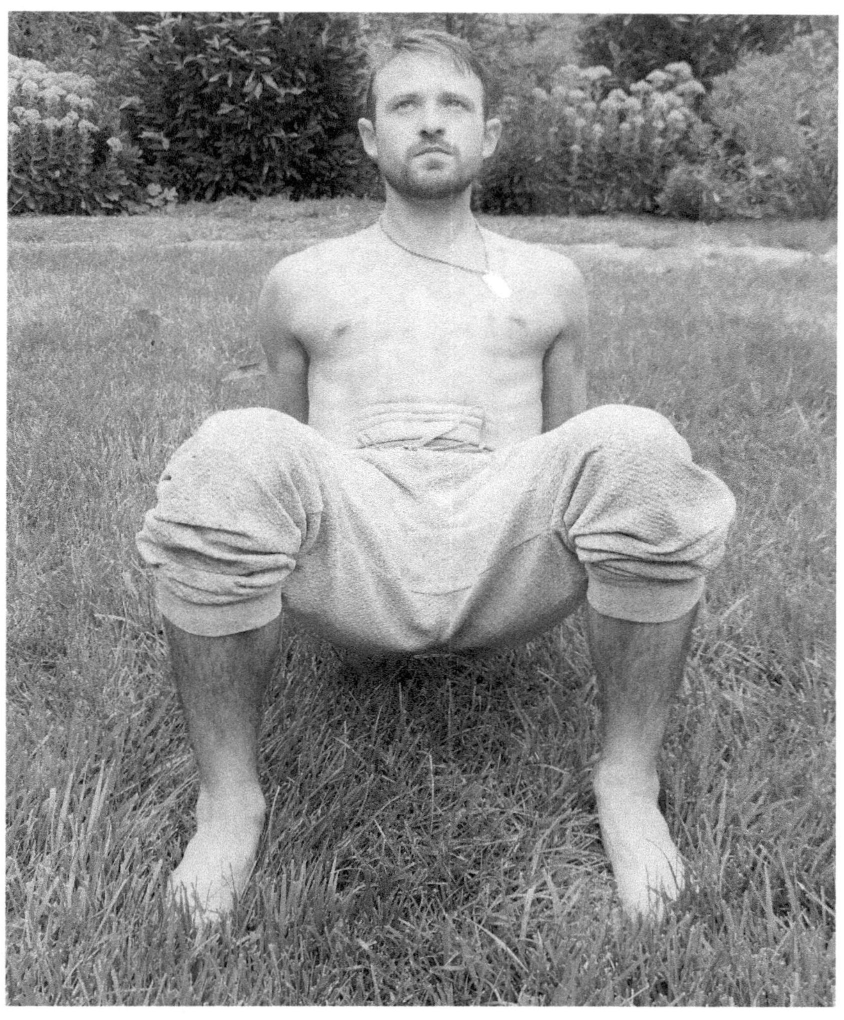

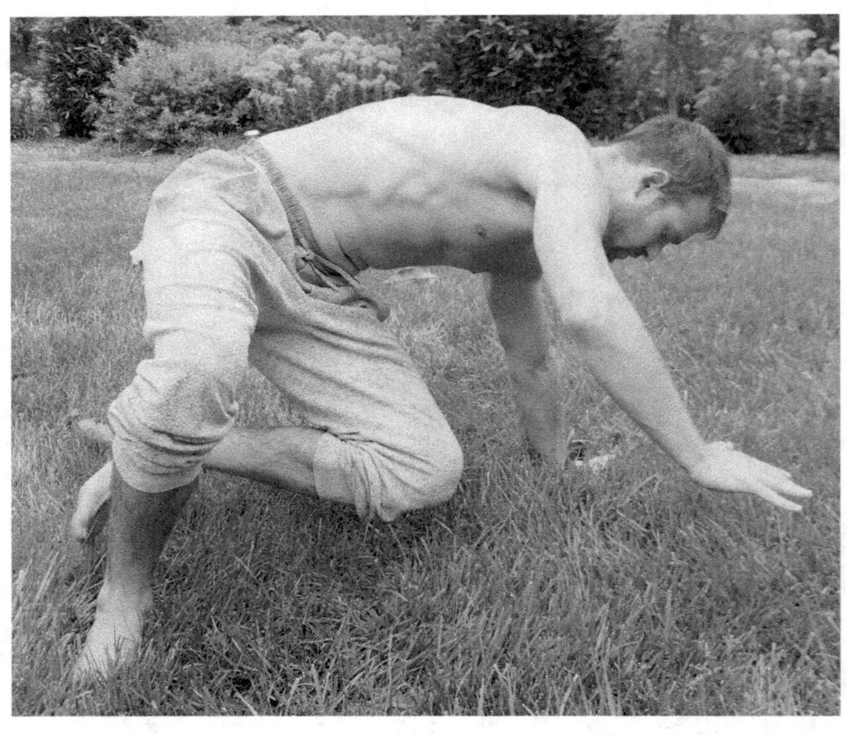

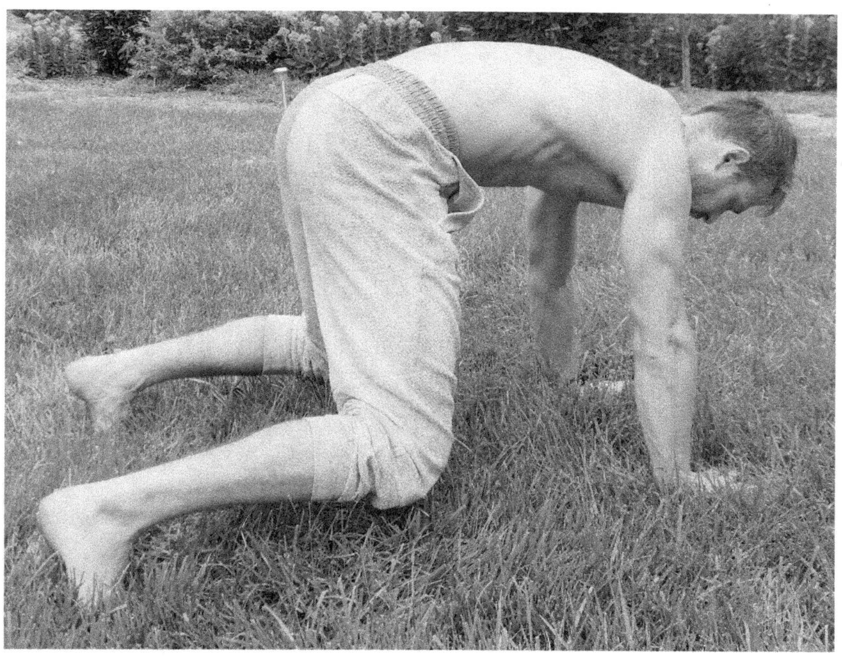

6. Scorpion Reach: Maintain a quadruped position. Lifting your hips, reach your right leg and circle over and across to the left side of your body. 3

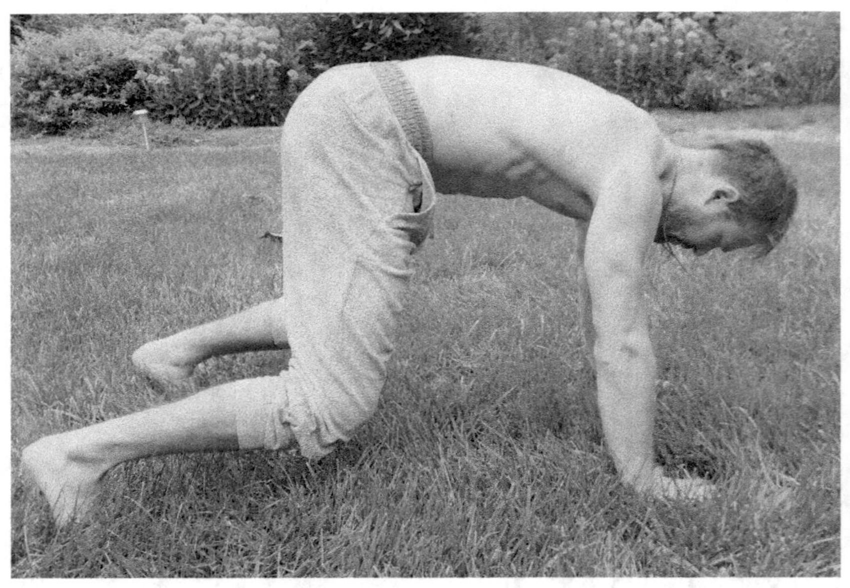

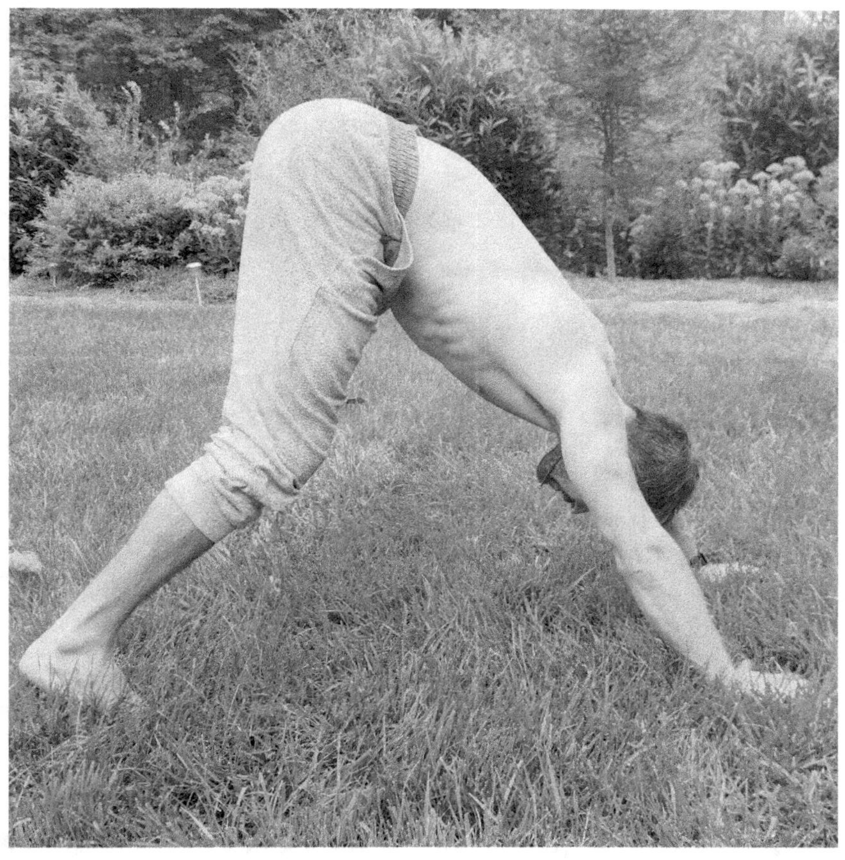

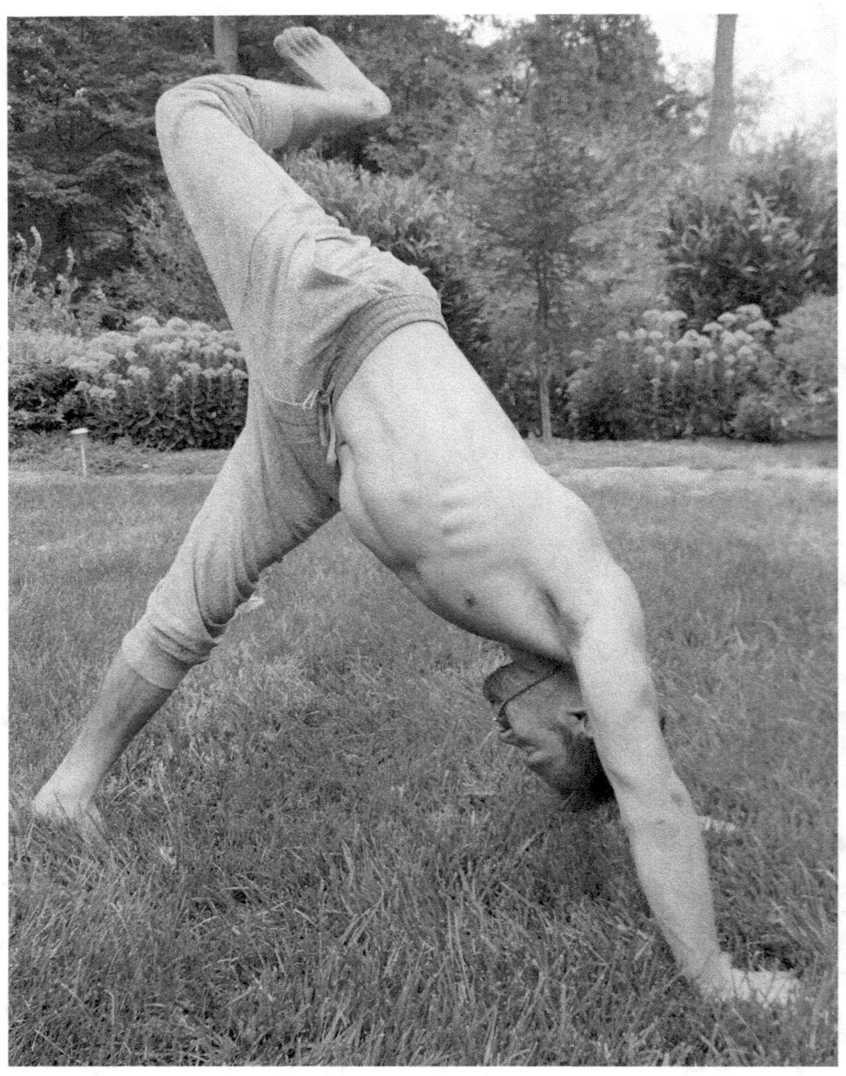

7. Crab Walk: Sit with feet flat and hands behind you, fingers pointing backward. Lift your hips and walk backward, staying in a tabletop position. Weight should be balanced, pressing through the shoulders with your butt in the middle of where your hands and feet are. Lifting your left hand and right foot, walk forward. Alternate hands and feet to progress.

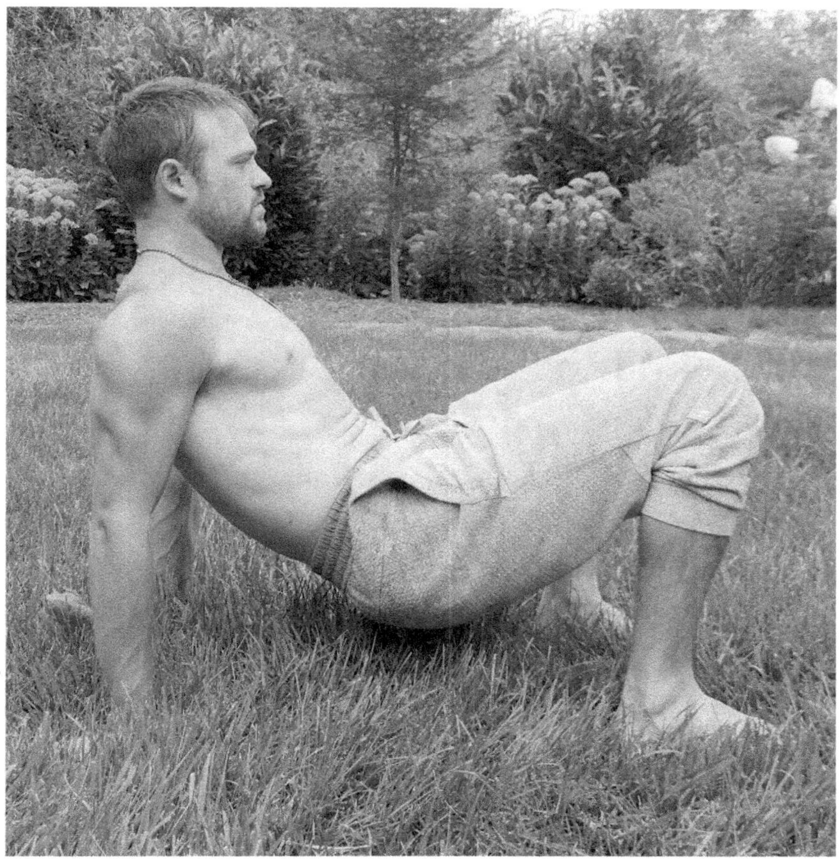

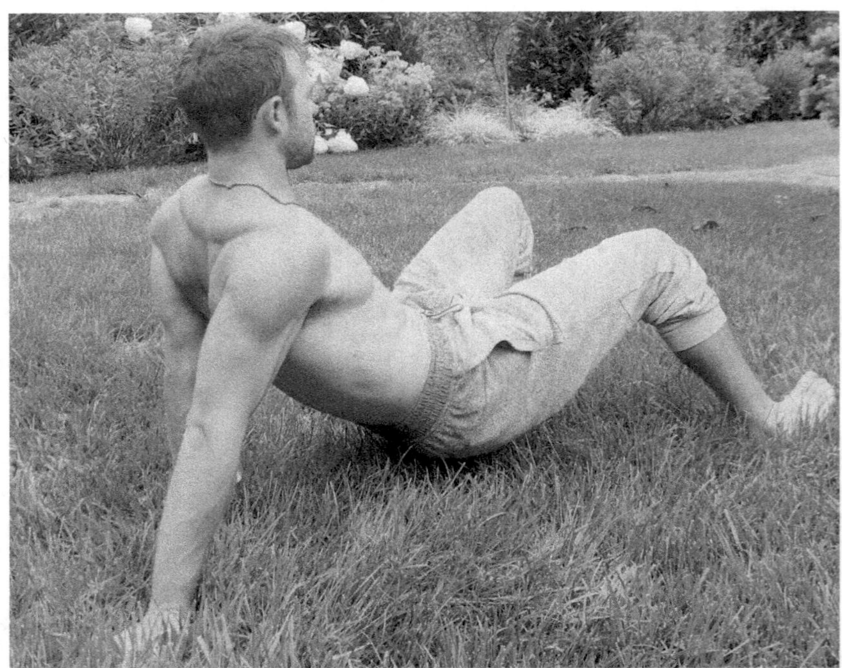

8. Gorilla Walk: Stand with feet wide apart and squat down. Walk forward in a squat position, keeping hands on the ground. Same leg, same hand moves at the same time.

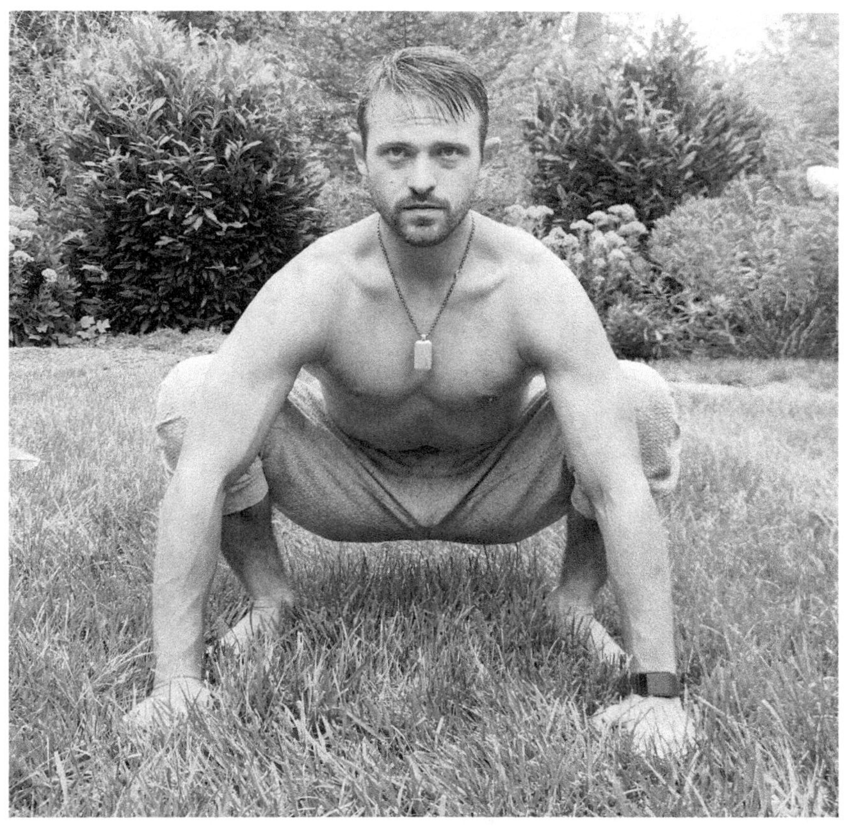

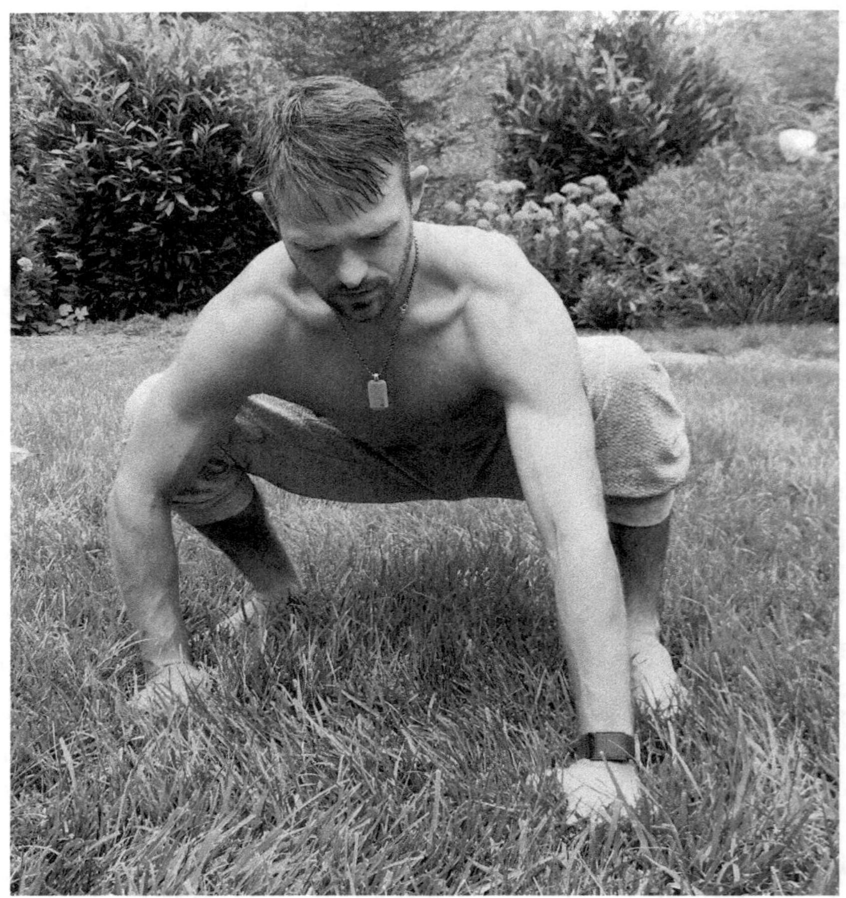

9. Lateral Traveling Beast: Start in a quadruped position and move laterally, keeping hips low and alternating the leading hand and foot.

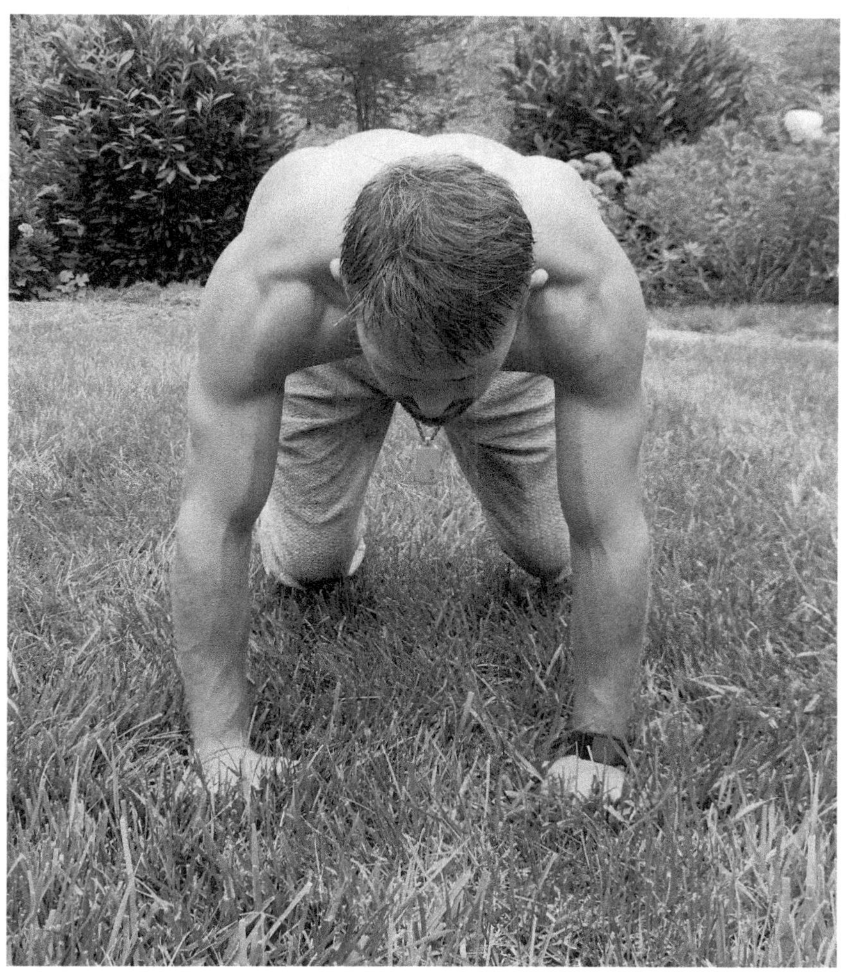

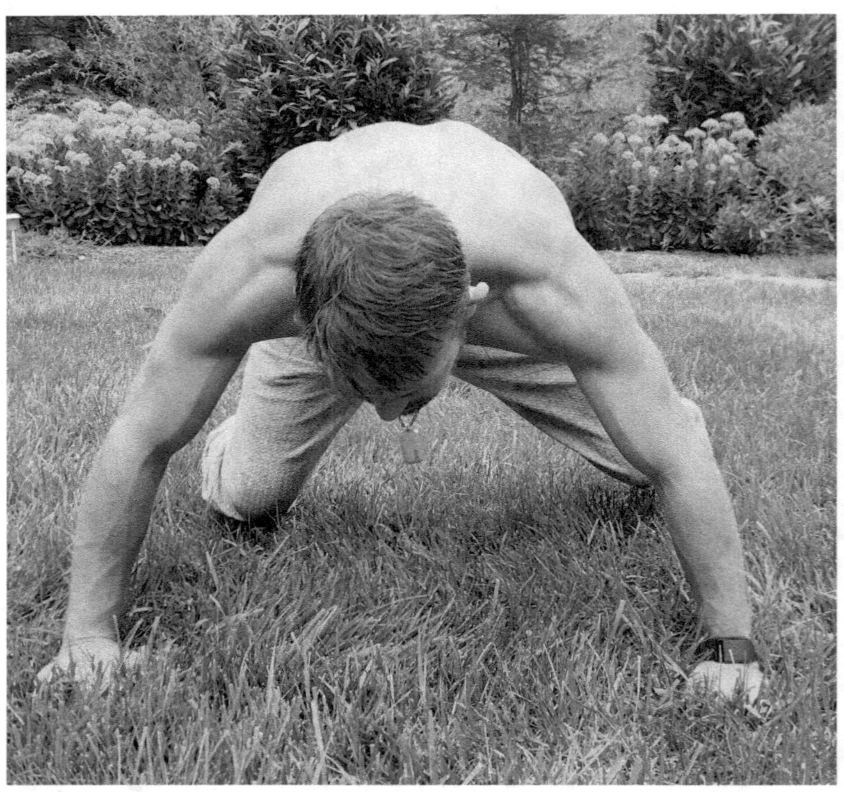

10. Frog Jump: Stand with feet wide apart and squat down. Jump forward as if leaping like a frog, then return to the starting position.

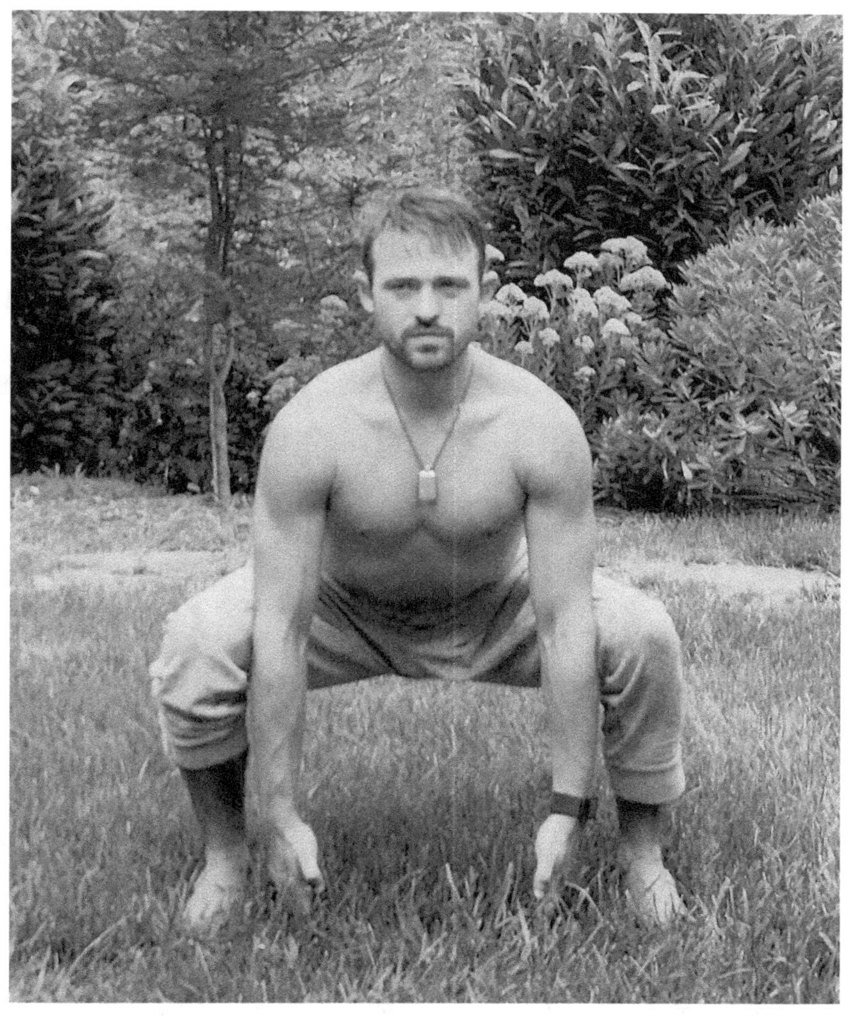

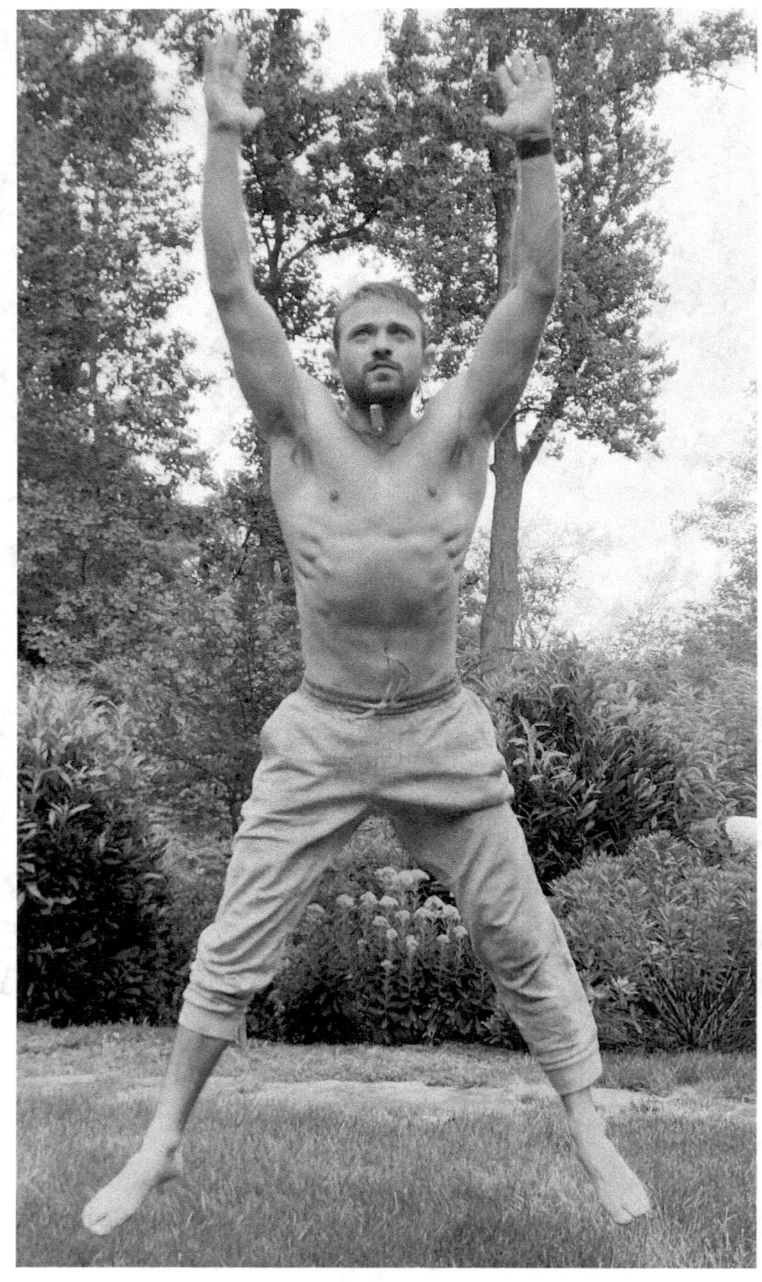

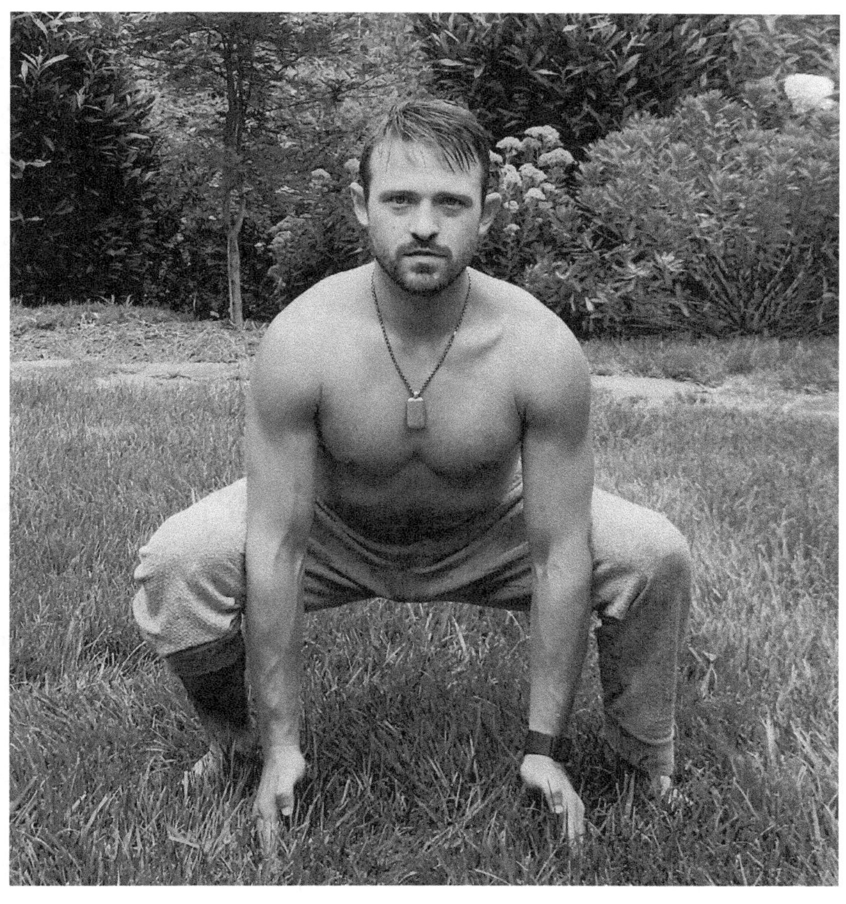

14

5-Day Animal Flow PREP Plan

Day 1: Beast Crawl and Crab Reach

Both the Beast Crawl and Crab Reach exercises are excellent for enhancing overall strength, stability, and coordination. They engage multiple muscle groups and challenge your body in unique ways, making them valuable additions to your fitness routine. Always remember to perform these exercises on a comfortable surface and with proper form to prevent injuries and get the most out of your workout.

DAY 2: Ape Reach and Bear Crawl

The Ape Reach and Bear Crawl exercises are fantastic for developing functional strength, agility, and mobility. They mimic the movements of their animal namesakes, tapping into the primal energy within us. Incorporate these exercises into your fitness routine for a fun and challenging full-body workout that will leave you feeling strong and agile like the creatures of the wild. As with any exercise, always prioritize proper form and listen to your body to avoid injury and maximize the benefits of your workout.

DAY 3: Underswitch and Scorpion Reach

Explore fluid transitions and mesmerizing stretches with the Underswitch and Scorpion Reach. Experience the seamless flow of movement as you switch between handstands and side planks with grace and ease. Embrace the beauty of the scorpion reach, reaching across your body like the majestic creature itself. Unleash your inner creativity and immerse yourself in the art of mindful movement. Both the Underswitch and Scorpion Reach exercises are excellent for building core strength, stability, and flexibility. They engage multiple muscle groups and require coordination and control, making them valuable additions to your workout routine. As with any exercise, be mindful of your body's limitations and modify the movements as needed to ensure safety and optimal results. Enjoy the challenge and embrace the primal movements that awaken the adventurer within!

DAY 4: Gorilla Walk and Frog Jump

Both the Gorilla Walk and Frog Jump exercises are dynamic and powerful movements that engage multiple muscle groups and elevate your heart rate. They promote lower body strength, endurance, and coordination while adding a fun and adventurous element to your workout routine. Always remember to perform these exercises on a safe and comfortable surface, and listen to your body to avoid overexertion or injury. Get ready to unleash your primal energy and experience the excitement of moving like a gorilla and leaping like a frog!

DAY 5: Lateral Traveling Beast and Crab Walk

The Traveling Beast and Crab Walk exercises are excellent for enhancing agility, coordination, and overall body strength. They add a sense of adventure to your workout routine and encourage you to embrace your inner beast and crab. As with any exercise, focus on maintaining proper form and listen to your body to prevent injury. Feel the freedom of movement and let these primal-inspired exercises take you on a journey to discover the untamed spirit within you!

15

5-Day Animal Flow Workout Plan

This 5-day routine will take you from beginner to intermediate levels, empowering you to explore your full potential through the art of Animal Flow.

Day 1: Beginner Flow

1. Beast Crawl - 3 sets of 10 meters

2. Crab Reach - 3 sets of 8 reps (each side)

3. Ape Reach - 3 sets of 10 reps (each side)

4. Bear Crawl - 3 sets of 10 meters

5. Underswitch - 3 sets of 8 reps (each side)

Day 2: Core and Balance

1. Scorpion Reach - 3 sets of 10 reps (each side)

2. Crab Walk - 3 sets of 10 meters

3. Gorilla Walk - 3 sets of 10 meters

4. Traveling Beast - 3 sets of 8 meters (each side)

5. Frog Jump - 3 sets of 10 reps

Day 3: Intermediate Flow

1. Beast Crawl - 4 sets of 10 meters

2. Crab Reach - 4 sets of 8 reps (each side)

3. Ape Reach - 4 sets of 10 reps (each side)

4. Bear Crawl - 4 sets of 10 meters

5. Underswitch - 4 sets of 8 reps (each side)

6. Scorpion Reach - 3 sets of 10 reps (each side)

7. Crab Walk - 3 sets of 10 meters

Day 4: Total Body Challenge

1. Gorilla Walk - 4 sets of 10 meters

2. Frog Jump - 4 sets of 10 reps

3. Traveling Beast - 4 sets of 8 meters (each side)

4. Crab Walk - 4 sets of 10 meters

5. Scorpion Reach - 4 sets of 10 reps (each side)

6. Beast Crawl - 3 sets of 10 meters

Day 5: Flexibility and Mobility

1. Ape Reach - 4 sets of 10 reps (each side)

2. Crab Reach - 4 sets of 8 reps (each side)

3. Bear Crawl - 4 sets of 10 meters

4. Underswitch - 4 sets of 8 reps (each side)

5. Scorpion Reach - 4 sets of 10 reps (each side)

6. Frog Jump - 3 sets of 10 reps

Remember to warm up before each session and cool down with gentle stretches afterward. Listen to your body, and progress at a pace that suits your fitness level. Stay consistent and have fun exploring the exciting world of Animal Flow!

16

Safety Guidelines for a Thriving Primal Flow Practice:

In the pursuit of embracing Primal Flow and unlocking the hidden secrets of nature's fitness code, safety stands as a cornerstone of your journey. As you immerse yourself in the captivating world of natural movements, it's essential to prioritize your well-being to ensure a successful and injury-free experience.

Start Slowly and Progress Gradually: Rome wasn't built in a day, and neither is a thriving Primal Flow practice. Begin your journey with simple movements and gradually increase the intensity. Embrace patience and allow your body to adapt to new challenges, one step at a time.

Proper Warm-up and Cool-down: Before delving into the heart of Primal Flow, take a moment to prepare your body with a dynamic warm-up. Gentle stretches and mobility exercises will prime your muscles and joints, reducing the risk of injury. Likewise, honor your body with a soothing cool-down after your practice, fostering flexibility and promoting recovery.

Pay Attention to Form: The essence of Primal Flow lies in the quality of your movement. Focus on proper form during each exercise to maximize its benefits and minimize the risk of injury. When in doubt, seek guidance from a fitness professional or refer to instructional resources.

Mindful Breathing: Embrace the union of breath and movement during your Primal Flow practice. With each exercise, synchronize your breath, inhaling deeply during the preparatory phase and exhaling as you execute the movement. This mindful connection will enhance your mind-body awareness and elevate your practice to new heights.

Use Proper Footwear (or None at All): When engaging in ground-contact exercises, consider minimalist shoes or opt for the liberating experience of barefoot training. Both options enhance your connection to the earth, allowing for more natural foot movement.

Modify for Your Fitness Level: Primal Flow welcomes enthusiasts of all fitness levels. Don't shy away from modifying exercises to suit your abilities. If a movement feels overly challenging, choose a regression that aligns with your current strength and mobility.

Respect Your Limits: Pushing your limits is crucial for growth, but know when to draw the line. Avoid pushing yourself to the point of discomfort or pain. Listen to your body, and if needed, take rest days to facilitate recovery and prevent overtraining.

Mind the Environment: Nature's playground offers a captivating backdrop for Primal Flow, but always remain mindful of your surroundings. Select a safe and clear space, free from potential obstacles or hazards, to fully immerse yourself in the experience.

Stay Hydrated: Hydration is key to sustaining peak performance during your Primal Flow sessions. Keep a trusty water bottle by your side and remember to replenish your body with plenty of fluids.

Listen to Your Body: Amid the exhilaration of Primal Flow, remember to stay attuned to your body's cues. If a movement feels uncomfortable or painful, stop the exercise and consult with a professional if needed.

Incorporate Rest and Recovery: The pursuit of optimal fitness requires both effort and rest. Embrace a well-rounded approach that incorporates rest and recovery to nurture your body and mind after intense workouts.

Incorporate Cross-Training: While Primal Flow offers a comprehensive fitness experience, embrace cross-training to diversify your routine and prevent overuse injuries. Activities like swimming, yoga, or hiking complement Primal Flow, allowing you to thrive from a spectrum of physical challenges.

In the spirit of Primal Flow, may you embark on your fitness journey with a heart brimming with excitement and a mind vigilant with safety and effectiveness. By adhering to these guidelines and tips, you pave the way for a flourishing Primal Flow practice, one that elevates your physical potential while honoring your body's innate wisdom.

17

THANK YOU

Thank you for embarking on this transformative journey with "The Hidden Secrets of Primal Flow: Unleashing Nature's Fitness Code." I hope this book has ignited a newfound passion for natural and functional fitness, reconnecting you with the primal wisdom that resides within. Embracing Primal Flow can lead to profound changes in your physical, mental, and emotional well-being, empowering you to live life to its fullest.

If you found value in these pages and enjoyed your experience with "The Hidden Secrets of Primal Flow," I kindly invite you to leave a review on Amazon. Your feedback not only encourages other readers to embark on this empowering journey but also helps spread the message of nature-inspired fitness to a broader audience. Together, we can inspire a movement toward mindful movement and unleash the untamed power that lies within each of us.

Thank you once again for being part of this incredible adventure. May your path be filled with boundless vitality, strength, and a deep connection to the world around you. Keep flowing with the pulse of nature, and remember that the wild essence of movement is forever within your reach. All the love, all the power.

18

RESOURCES

https://www.thefitfoodielife.com/the-benefits-of-primal-movement/#:~:text=For%20starters%2C%20it%20improves%20joint,great%20for%20improving%20cardiovascular%20health

Heather. The Benefits of Primal Movement: Why Everyone Should Try It - The Fit Foodie Life. The Fit Foodie Life. Published February 1, 2023. https://www.thefitfoodielife.com/the-benefits-of-primal-movement/#:~:text=For%20starters%2C%20it%20improves%20joint,great%20for%20improving%20cardiovascular%20health

https://www.dailyom.com/journal/what-is-primal-movement-learn-about-it-s-benefits-exercises-and-more/
https://theeverygirl.com/primal-movement/

https://www.dailyom.com/journal/what-is-primal-movement-learn-about-it-s-benefits-exercises-and-more/ https://theeverygirl.com/pri

mal-movement/.

https://www.gcc.edu/Home/News-Archive/News-Article/buxtons-exercise-science-study-finds-primal-workout-benefits

Hildebrand N. Buxton's exercise science study finds primal workout benefits. *Grove City College*. https://www.gcc.edu/Home/News-Archi ve/News-Article/buxtons-exercise-science-study-finds-primal-worko ut-benefits. Published November 29, 2021.

https://www.chattersource.com/article/animal-flow/

De Alba S. Why Primal Movement Is All The Rage In Fitness [The New CrossFit] | ChatterSource. ChatterSource. Published August 3, 2021. https://www.chattersource.com/article/animal-flow/

https://www.movnat.com/the-roots-of-methode-naturelle/

Admin. The roots of "Methode Naturelle" *MovNat: Natural Movement Fitness*. Published online June 13, 2016. https://www.movnat.com/the-roots-of-methode-naturelle/

https://www.saturdayeveningpost.com/2019/08/does-our-primitive -survival-instinct-still-work-in-the-21st-century/

Taylor J PhD. Does our primitive survival instinct still work in the 21st century? *The Saturday Evening Post*. Published online August 28, 2019.

https://www.saturdayeveningpost.com/2019/08/does-our-primitive-survival-instinct-still-work-in-the-21st-century/

https://zahieradams.medium.com/natures-footprints-exploring-the-remarkable-feet-of-the-huaorani-tribe-32e100583a90

Adams Z. Nature's footprints: Exploring the remarkable feet of the Huaorani Tribe. *Medium*. https://zahieradams.medium.com/natures-footprints-exploring-the-remarkable-feet-of-the-huaorani-tribe-32e100583a90. Published June 15, 2023.

https://experiencelife.lifetime.life/article/animal-flow-fitness/

Life Time. Animal flow fitness. Experience Life. Published May 31, 2022. https://experiencelife.lifetime.life/article/animal-flow-fitness/

www.ingramcontent.com/pod-product-compliance
Lightning Source LLC
Chambersburg PA
CBHW070957250726
48663CB00002B/266